Language Matters

*Appropriate Language Guide
for Supporting People in Distress*

Anthony Smith and Melissa Raven

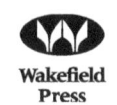

Wakefield Press

Wakefield Press
16 Rose Street
Mile End
South Australia 5031
www.wakefieldpress.com.au

First published 2024

Copyright © Anthony Smith and Melissa Raven, 2024

All rights reserved. This book is copyright. Apart from
any fair dealing for the purposes of private study, research,
criticism or review, as permitted under the Copyright Act,
no part may be reproduced without written permission.
Enquiries should be addressed to the publisher.

Edited by Julia Beaven, Wakefield Press
Typeset by Michael Deves

ISBN 978 1 92304 269 8

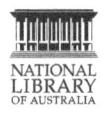

A catalogue record for this book is available from the National Library of Australia

Wakefield Press thanks Coriole Vineyards for continued support

Contents

Preface		**vii**
1	Choosing language that helps rather than harms	**1**
2	Distress and suicidality	**3**
3	Problematic terms	**9**
4	Risk factors and protective factors	**19**
5	The spectrum of suicide prevention activity	**23**
6	Understanding key concepts about research and practice	**28**
Acknowledgements		**37**
Notes		**38**

Wakefield Press

Language Matters

Anthony Smith has established a national profile in Australian suicide prevention. He is the author of *Default Depression: How we now interpret distress as mental illness* (Wakefield Press) and co-author of the 'Situational Approach' papers and other suicide prevention papers and research. Anthony has a long history of activity in a range of suicide prevention settings. He is currently an investigator working with the Critical and Ethical Mental Health (CEMH) group at the University of Adelaide on a major federally funded suicide prevention research project.

Melissa Raven is a research fellow with the Critical and Ethical Mental Health group at the University of Adelaide. She originally qualified as a clinical psychologist, and subsequently completed a masters in epidemiology and a PhD critically analysing claims and evidence about depression and antidepressants. Her mental health research and advocacy is informed by a strong social determinants perspective and a strong critical orientation, which she applies to a range of topics, including suicide prevention, workplace mental health, (over)diagnosis, (inappropriate) prescribing, and financial/nonfinancial conflicts of interest in mental health and the broader health/welfare arena.

By the same authors

Default Depression   Anthony Smith

Preface

There is increasing concern about excessive medicalisation of common human behaviours and emotions. Too often, distress is interpreted as symptomatic of mental illness. Diagnoses of mental disorders, and prescriptions of antidepressants and other psychotropic drugs, have increased dramatically in recent decades, facilitated by ever-increasing funding for mental health and suicide prevention. Despite this, suicide deaths are continuing to increase, suggesting that medicalisation of distress may not be the answer. Policies and practices driving this medicalisation are now well-established, not only in the health/welfare system, but also throughout every sector of the community, including the workplace, education, sport, and media.

A key driver of medicalisation is the use of language and terminology that promotes a narrow clinical approach at the expense of considering broader causes of distress. Language matters. The use of appropriate language is crucial to responding helpfully to people in distress.

The current clinical approach relies on pathologising and potentially disempowering concepts and language, such as mental disorder and mental illness, particularly 'depression' and 'anxiety disorder'.

This booklet, *Language Matters: Appropriate Language Guide for Supporting People in Distress* presents alternative, more helpful language. It is informed by the Situational Approach, a new conceptual framework for considering and responding to human distress. The Situational Approach is underpinned by recognition of the need to acknowledge and address wider issues that contribute to distress (including unemployment, poverty, relationship problems, and grief).

Language Matters is a resource that addresses specific language and terminology in common usage in the mental health/suicide prevention sector as well as throughout our community. It provides a practical set of terms and definitions for compassionately assisting people experiencing distress.

1
Choosing language that helps rather than harms

Language matters. The words and phrases we use can shape our experience and the experience of others. The use of appropriate language is crucial to facilitating appropriate support to people in distress.

This booklet is part language guide, part glossary. It discusses language that is useful and language that is problematic, to provide guidance to health/welfare workers, and anyone with an interest in mental health and suicide prevention. It provides a practical set of terms and definitions for dealing with the distress related to a broad spectrum of human difficulties experienced by many people and frequently encountered by practitioners in the suicide prevention/ mental health field.

Despite the good intentions of many people working in suicide prevention and/or mental health, including workplace mental health (WMH), some of the terminology in common usage is problematic and unhelpful.

Pathologising language, using terms such as 'disorder' and 'illness', and particularly diagnostic labels such as 'depression' and 'anxiety disorder', is far from innocuous. It can, in fact, be harmful. Such language can be derogatory; it can increase stigma and social marginalisation, and it can contribute to depression and anxiety disorder. It can also transform the way people see and define themselves, often for a lifetime. In particular, it can disempower people, making them feel helpless and reliant on expert intervention. On the other hand, providing a succinct, non-clinical description with appropriate language may be reassuring, with less risk of adverse negative effects.

Language Matters is a companion to the book *Default Depression: How we now interpret distress as mental illness,* published in Adelaide by Wakefield Press in 2023. It discusses problematic language commonly used to discuss distress, and provides more appropriate terms as an alternative.

This guide and the *Default Depression* book are informed by the Situational Approach,[1] a new conceptual framework for how we can consider and respond to human distress. The Situational Approach focuses on situational distress rather than mental disorders. It is underpinned by recognition of the need to acknowledge and address wider issues that contribute to distress (including unemployment, poverty, relationship problems, and grief). It has been developed to encourage appropriate, competent, caring, supportive responses to individuals in distress.

The Situational Approach is a significant departure from the current medical framework for suicide prevention and mental health, with its emphasis on illness and the use of pathologising language.

In general, we recommend that people should avoid the use of clinical labels to refer to other people. There are exceptions. Sometimes people with a supporting role (including health/welfare workers and human resources [HR] staff) need to use diagnostic labels for various purposes, such as providing detail for health insurance claims.

2
Distress and suicidality

Distress is a major contributor to suicidality, and it is important to understand this relationship and use appropriate terminology. Some of the terms below come from the Situational Approach. Other terms are already in common usage, but are clarified here to facilitate a compassionate, less medicalised approach to dealing with distress. The definitions are not exhaustive, and are likely to evolve as the Situational Approach becomes more firmly established as a conceptual framework in the mental health/suicide prevention sector.

Table 1. Key Situational Approach terms

Key term	Explanation/discussion
situational distress	Situational distress encompasses a significantly challenging or troubling experience of thoughts, emotions, bodily sensations, and/or behaviours associated with difficult life events, such as bereavement, health problems, relationship breakdown, financial problems, or occupational difficulties. This distress may significantly overlap with many of the symptoms usually taken to suggest mental disorders (particularly depression and anxiety disorders).[2]
	The conceptual basis for situational distress acknowledges social determinants of health and welfare, such as unemployment, and financial and relationship difficulties, as having a key role as causal factors in distress. However, sometimes, even in cases of acute distress, there are no obvious causal social factors. Nevertheless, the situational context remains a vitally important consideration. Regardless of the causal factors involved, people in significant distress need their situational context – including family context, finances, health/mental health and availability of community support services – to be considered as a priority for appropriate responses and support.

Key term	Explanation/discussion
psychological distress	Psychological distress refers to patterns of psychological and emotional discomfort and general unpleasant feelings and emotions. It is an umbrella term to describe some common interrelated problems, including stress, depression, anxiety, and suicidal thoughts.
	Psychological distress should not be automatically presumed to be a mental disorder. It is often associated with external and internal factors such as: workplace stress, financial difficulties, bullying and abuse, interpersonal difficulties, bereavement, lack of sleep, use of drugs or alcohol, and/or physical illness. The distress associated with such factors can be compounded by thoughts and feelings of powerlessness, which can impair cognitive functioning,[3] including making it harder for people to engage in constructive problem-solving.
high-intensity psychological distress	High-intensity psychological distress refers to serious psychological and emotional distress, which may necessitate active support, for example clinical intervention and/or other support.
	This level of distress usually significantly impairs a person's ability to function on a day-to-day basis and interferes with their usual mental, emotional, or social capacity, and their experience of feeling capable and competent.
	Persistent distress of this intensity often requires more than a person's own coping ability, lifestyle adjustments, and support of friends and family. At least initially, it may require thoughtful observation and reflective assessment by a health professional (such as a GP, psychologist, or, in some cases, a psychiatrist), who may also suggest appropriate psychotherapy (psychological therapy).
	The term 'high-intensity psychological distress' is a less pathologising alternative to commonly used but ambiguous and potentially disempowering terms such as *mental disorder* or *mental illness*.

People suffering high-intensity psychological distress may be at significantly elevated risk of suicide.[4] This distress is often associated with difficult social and financial circumstances that may precipitate or entrench a state of despair or hopelessness. Some of these people may benefit from timely professional support, but it is important not to assume that the support of mental health professionals is always necessary or appropriate or helpful. Furthermore, the assumption that

Distress and suicidality

mental health professionals have the solutions deflects attention from responses that address situational factors.

There is a situational context relevant to every suicide death, and every suicide attempt. Often there is significant situational distress in the preceding days, weeks, months, or even years. Unfortunately, the dominant focus on mental disorders as the cause of suicide often deflects attention from situational distress and its causes. This occurs both in relation to understanding suicides that have occurred and in relation to suicide prevention.

Extensive research shows that many people who kill themselves have no history of mental disorders.[5] Furthermore, regardless of their mental health history, they are usually impacted by difficult social circumstances.[6] The majority of people who kill themselves have been in circumstances likely to cause enormous stress in their lives, such as unemployment – the majority of all suicide deaths in Australia from 2002 to 2013 were people of working age who were not employed at the time of their death.[7] However, the relationship between unemployment, distress, and suicide risk is complex, because distress from other causes can also impact on the ability to hold a job. It is crucial that social determinants such as employment be considered as a priority in current and future suicide prevention planning and initiatives.

Many people who die by suicide have recently engaged with mental health professionals, including GPs.[8] Unfortunately, research into this issue has not clarified the extent to which current stress/distress was specifically discussed or addressed.

Men are less likely than women to seek formal mental health support.[9] However, it is important not to assume that simply encouraging men to seek such support will reduce their suicide risk. Significant concerns have been raised about the appropriateness and effectiveness of services generally to meet the needs of men. Furthermore, there is insufficient attention paid to other ways that men might seek help when they are troubled.[10]

Despite the important role of adverse life events in suicide, much of the current approach to suicide prevention continues to focus narrowly and unhelpfully on mental disorders. Limiting preventive strategies to those built upon the presumption that suicide is generally caused by mental disorders will simply not help many, perhaps the majority, of people at risk of suicide. This is not the only risk. There is also evidence that inappropriate support can discourage people from seeking help again.[11]

Effective suicide prevention requires strategies that are non-pathologising and are part of a broader, more encompassing approach that takes account of social determinants.

Table 2. Suicide-related terms

suicidality	Suicidality refers to a range of states and behaviours, from 'suicidal ideation' (having thoughts about suicide and/or being dead), through planning death by suicide and/or attempting suicide.
	It is quite common for people to have serious thoughts about taking their own life. In 2020–21, 1 in 6 (approximately 3.3 million) Australians aged 16–85 reported having had experienced serious thoughts about taking their own life at some point in their lives.[26] People who experience suicidal thoughts and/or behaviours (suicidality) are at greater risk of completing suicide.[27] However, it is important to understand that, although people who experience suicidal ideation and even those who make suicide plans are at increased risk of suicide attempts, very few go on to kill themselves.[28]
	There is a gender paradox to suicidality; despite the much higher rate of completed male suicides, females have higher rates of suicidal ideation, suicide plans and (incomplete) attempts.[29]
	As with distress more generally, it is crucial to consider the situational context of people who are suicidal.
suicide	Suicide refers to death resulting from deliberate self-injury or other physical self-harm (e.g. poisoning), with the intention of dying.
attempted suicide	Attempted suicide refers to deliberate self-injury or other physical self-harm (e.g. poisoning), with the intention of dying. Although there is some overlap between people who attempt but do not complete suicide and those who do complete suicide, these groups are characterised by significant demographic and clinical differences.[30] Again, few who have attempted suicide go on to complete it, and there is some evidence[31] that many suicide deaths, perhaps the majority, occur on the first attempt.

Language Matters

self-harm	Self-harm refers to deliberate self-injury or other physical self-harm, such as cutting, burning, self-poisoning, or overdosing on drugs (including prescription medications) and/or alcohol.
	Self-harm is common, and not only among teenagers.[32] However, it is crucial to note that, in most cases, self-harm is not an attempt at suicide and does not lead to suicide, but is rather a way of coping with unmanageable feelings.[33]
	The relationship between suicide and self-harm is complicated. People with a history of self-harm are at considerably higher risk of suicide.[34]
	Most cases of self-harm occur in females, as do most cases of attempted but incomplete suicide; but most suicide deaths occur in males.[35] In many cases of self-harm, there is a history of behavioural difficulties, substance misuse, and family, social and psychological problems.[36] None of this should be uncritically presumed to indicate a mental disorder.
	An attempt should always be made to understand what underpins self-harm, whether or not the intention is suicide.

3
Problematic terms

To facilitate more appropriate language use, this section discusses some of the more problematic terms in common usage, and offers some options for alternative language.

Some of the problematic terms might be appropriate in a clinical or administrative setting, but otherwise can deflect attention from situational factors causing stress. Clinical diagnoses can overshadow other problems in people's lives and can narrow the range of interventions that are considered.

As stated, we recommend that, where possible, non-clinicians should avoid the use of clinical labels to refer to other people.

Table 3. Problematic terms and recommended alternatives

Problematic terms	Recommended use, alternative terms
depression The term 'depression' is highly ambiguous. It confuses and conflates normal (albeit sometimes distressing and highly challenging) human experience with pathological categorisations, and reinforces medicalisation/pathologisation. The experience of being human can sometimes be acutely distressing, even overwhelming and debilitating. Nevertheless, such experience does not necessarily constitute a diagnosable mental disorder, and in fact is often a normal response to stressful events such as financial difficulties, workplace problems, or housing problems.	'distress', 'psychological/emotional distress' When relevant, use descriptive language that says more about the person's experience – for example, loss of meaning in work, money worries, 'loneliness' or 'grief'.
anxiety The terms 'anxiety' and 'anxiety disorder' can be ambiguous. In particular, 'anxiety' is often used inappropriately as a synonym/euphemism for 'anxiety disorder'. The word 'anxiety' needs to be reclaimed in its original meaning. Anxiety is a natural human state, experienced by everyone at times. It is a normal and healthy reaction to stress that has both psychological features (e.g. fear, irritability) and physiological features (e.g. sweating). Anxiety should not be automatically assumed to be a symptom/indication of a mental disorder.	'stress', 'distress', 'anxiety about …', 'worry' It may often be helpful to refer to the specific cause(s) of stress (e.g. worry about potential redundancy, anxiety about rising interest rates and mortgage payments, anxiety about family problems).
anxiety disorder Anxiety levels may become overwhelming for some people, with a debilitating impact on their daily lives. If this is a chronic problem, meeting the diagnostic criteria for an anxiety disorder, people may require clinical treatment.	'anxiety', 'ongoing anxiety', 'chronic anxiety', 'debilitating anxiety', 'serious anxiety' Refer to a person as having an anxiety disorder only if it has been diagnosed by a doctor, and only mention it when it is relevant.

Problematic terms

Problematic terms	Recommended use, alternative terms
mental illness/mental disorder/psychiatric disorder As with *'depression'*, these terms are highly ambiguous; perpetuate medicalisation/pathologisation.	'distress', 'situational distress' It is generally better to avoid these highly medicalised terms (mental illness/mental disorder/psychiatric disorder), or at least to explain the specific meaning of the terms as you are using them (e.g. when discussing rates of mental disorders reported in surveys, note that most cases are likely to be mild). When engaging with individual people in distress, avoid terms such as mental illness altogether. Instead, discuss the issues causing distress, for example an excessively demanding workload, or relationship problems.
mental health 'Mental health' is an ambiguous term, and is often used as a euphemism for mental illness. Most importantly, it detracts attention from the broader context and factors affecting an individual's distress; serves to reinforce the medicalisation of distress, and limits the scope of interventions to mental health professionals (including GPs).	'wellbeing', 'health and wellbeing', 'personal/psychological/emotional wellbeing' 'social and emotional wellbeing' (SEWB) – a term commonly used by Aboriginal and Torres Strait Islander people (Indigenous Australians).[12]
mental health expert The term 'expert' as it applies to suicide prevention/mental health is problematic. Some of the most high-profile experts have, for decades, been strong advocates for a narrow medicalised approach to mental health. The problematic nature of the term 'mental health expert' is further compounded by the role of GPs, who provide the majority of mental health diagnosis and treatment.[13]	Describe by relevant occupation – for example, psychologist, psychiatrist, doctor, mental health nurse, or mental health researcher. Collectively, refer to as 'mental health professionals'.

Language Matters

Problematic terms	Recommended use, alternative terms
psychological injury	
The term 'psychological injury' is now commonly used in the workplace but is a highly problematic and often unhelpful term.	Avoid this term where possible. Alternative terms include 'situational distress', 'psychological distress', 'emotional distress'.
The word 'injury' generally means physical harm to the body – a discrete biological problem, often resulting in pain, caused by one or more specific physical incidents/exposures. Furthermore, physical injuries can often be resolved with medical treatment.	Very often, a more helpful approach would be to enquire about the cause(s) of the distress.
Psychological injury similarly implies a discrete psychological problem that can be resolved with treatment, regardless of context or cause. Furthermore, the emphasis is usually on mental disorders. This is clear in definitions such as: 'Psychological injury may include such disorders as depression, anxiety or post-traumatic stress disorder.'[14]	
The medicalisation of distress still prevails in the workplace, with workers' compensation legislation and policy for 'psychological injury'[15] or 'mental injury'[16] channelling workers along a medical pathway.	
The concept of psychological injury perpetuates the entrenched medicalised and individualised approach to workplace wellbeing. It has little or no relevance to situational distress caused by social and/or economic factors, and is not appropriate in the context of difficult workplace conditions.	

Problematic terms

Problematic terms	Recommended use, alternative terms
psychosocial hazards 'Psychosocial hazards' is a relatively new term in WMH, one of several terms intended to broaden the discussion about mental health beyond a narrow biomedical model. It is a key aspect of current workplace health and safety legislation and regulations. It is problematic for several reasons, and it still supports a medicalised and individualised approach to wellbeing. Workplace hazards are generally objects, activities, events, situations, or conditions that have the potential to harm people. Psychosocial hazards include long hours, shift-work, lack of job control, harassment, and bullying. Unfortunately, the distress caused by such hazards is generally interpreted as a mental disorder. For example, according to Safe Work Australia, 'A psychosocial hazard is anything that could cause psychological harm (e.g. harm someone's mental health)'.[17] Like 'psychological injury', this framing tends to channel workers along a medical pathway.[18] For example, according to Safe Work Australia, 'Psychological harm or injuries from psychosocial hazards include conditions such as anxiety, depression, post-traumatic stress disorder (PTSD) and sleep disorders'.[19] This reinforces a medicalised interpretation and response.	Avoid this term where possible. Depending on the context, alternative terms include 'situational stressors', 'stressors', 'stressful events', 'stressful circumstances'.
post-traumatic stress disorder (PTSD) PTSD refers to the debilitating state that a person may suffer following a relatively direct experience of a particularly harrowing event or series of events, such as being directly involved in acts of war or witnessing horrific accidents or instances of violence. PTSD is a well-recognised diagnostic category in the mental health arena, including WMH (particularly in relation to emergency workers) and has been in common usage for several decades. It has a much more specific meaning than trauma, and should not be used outside clinical settings.	'distress' caused by … Specify the cause of distress, e.g. following a sexual assault.

Language Matters

Problematic terms	Recommended use, alternative terms
trauma The concept of trauma is more general than PTSD, and it has found its way into common usage more recently. Trauma is generally used to describe ongoing distress/suffering following a distressing event or events, but, like medical labels, it oversimplifies the person's experience and ignores other determinants of distress. In engaging with people who may be suffering the effects of traumatic experience, ask questions that open up consideration of the context and impact of the trauma. Avoid a heavy focus on the traumatic event itself at the expense of the personal experience. Instead, acknowledge any suffering as a result of a traumatic experience and discuss possible ways to address the cause of the traumatic experience.	Ask questions about the context and impact of the traumatic events, such as: - *Did something bad happen?* - *Was that frightening for you?* - *How did you feel when that happened?* - *Were you injured or hurt in some way?* It might be appropriate to comment that a reported event sounds very difficult or challenging, or even (where warranted) awful/horrific. Regardless, it is important to address the person's need for support.
'living with' a mental disorder This commonly used term is considered respectful, but is problematic. In particular, it implies chronicity. It also implies that mental disorders dominate and define people, eclipsing other aspects of their lives. It can be inadvertently disempowering and patronising.	'experiencing distress', 'diagnosed with a mental disorder'

Problematic terms

Problematic terms	Recommended use, alternative terms
mental health literacy The concept of mental health literacy is a key theme in the mental health arena. It encourages people to interpret their experience, and other people's experience, particularly distress, through a mental illness lens, focusing on recognition and management and prevention of mental disorders.[20] Despite the inclusion of 'health' in the term, it traditionally focuses on knowledge and beliefs about mental ill-health.[21] It can encourage inappropriate pathologisation of common psychological experiences, which can become a self-fulfilling prophecy.[22] Furthermore, mental health literacy rarely if ever includes a consideration of social determinants of mental health (SDOMH). So people with employment/financial/housing problems are encouraged to focus inwardly, and potentially seek help for mental disorders, rather than seeking help for their employment/financial/housing problems.	It is more constructive to promote literacy about: • the primacy of relationships in determining wellbeing • the importance of being 'good at feelings' rather than aspiring to 'feeling good' • the importance of social determinants of health.
resilience The concept of resilience has become a favourite in mental health literature and training. Unfortunately, it is often used in a way that focuses responsibility on individuals to rely on personal resources/attributes to weather difficult times, deflecting attention from the social/economic/political factors that contribute to hardship.[23]	Acknowledge/comment on people's strengths where relevant.

Language Matters

Problematic terms	Recommended use, alternative terms
RUOK? (Are you OK?) Although this question/brand has become popular and heads a well-funded mental health campaign, it is problematic. Although well-intentioned, it is superficial and it may in fact exacerbate the difficulties some people face. People may not want to disclose their feelings, or may feel obliged to answer that they are okay when they are not. To engage in a helpful way with someone in distress may require well-trained interpersonal skills that not everyone possesses.	Seek a more open and dynamic engagement, for example: • *Has something happened?* • *How's it all going?* Where possible, personalise your comments, for example: • *I've noticed several times this week that you seem unhappy/stressed. Is something worrying you?*
treatment Emphasis on treatment is a key component of medicalisation. It presumes an identifiable biological problem that can be remedied with medical procedures. Treatment is often equated with drug treatment specifically, which is often claimed/implied to be a magic bullet.	'support', 'care' If possible, suggest an agency and or individual(s) who may be able to provide appropriate support, e.g. for financial or housing problems.
symptom Emphasis on symptoms is another key component of medicalisation and pathologisation.	Describe the behaviour or emotion as it is, e.g. 'distress', 'chronic tiredness', 'exhaustion'; 'feeling overloaded', 'feeling overwhelmed'.
patient Labelling people as patients is another key component of medicalisation. It also tends to objectify people.	When engaging with or referring to people in distress, it is generally best to avoid the term 'patient', unless referring to a specific engagement process with a medical/health practitioner/agency. It is generally better to refer to people as workers, students, parents, etc., when relevant.

Problematic terms

Problematic terms	Recommended use, alternative terms
consumer/mental health consumer/client Usually refers to a person who has been diagnosed with a mental disorder or disorders and often has ongoing engagement with the mental health system. This is problematic for several reasons. Firstly, 'consumer' is an economic term, implying a transactional relationship. Also, it implies a voluntary relationship, which is not always the case. Additionally, it creates a sense of disempowerment for some people who are engaged with the mental health system. Also, there can be confusion and conflict between the experiences of consumers and the experiences of carers, family, kin, and other supporters. In some cases, the interests of consumers are at odds with, or even in clear opposition to, the interests of carers.	'client', 'service user', 'patient', 'person with mental illness', 'person with lived experience', 'survivor', 'client', 'psychiatric survivor' NB: None of these terms are universally accepted or unproblematic. Ideally, wait to see what terms people use to refer to themselves, or ask them, if relevant.
client 'Client' overlaps with 'consumer', and has some similar issues. However, being a 'consumer' of mental health services is an identity that some people embrace, whereas being a 'client' is simply an objective label for a recipient of a service.	as above
lived experience 'Lived experience' generally refers to people with direct experience of challenges around suicide or attempted suicide, and/or diagnosis of mental illness and engagement with the mental health system. This direct experience may or may not apply to individuals who have attempted suicide and/or been diagnosed with a mental disorder, and/or their family members and close friends. Lived experience is an important consideration from both a direct supportive perspective and a broader social/political perspective,[24] but it can be ambiguous.	When using the term 'lived experience', be clear about whose 'lived experience' and what type of experience you are referring to.

Language Matters

Problematic terms	Recommended use, alternative terms
stigma In relation to mental illness, stigma is where a person's character or personality is denigrated or portrayed as blemished, or the person is devalued, based on beliefs about the symptoms of mental disorders. Stigma stereotypes and discredits people, and can lead to discrimination against people with mental disorders.	
destigmatisation Destigmatisation means a reduction in stigma. It is a common goal in mental health initiatives. Considerable effort has been made in recent decades to destigmatise mental illness by changing public attitudes towards people with mental disorders and mental health treatment (particularly use of medication such as antidepressants). Destigmatisation campaigns, however, have not been very successful. For example, a 2021 survey found that half of all Australian workers reported that they would not disclose a mental health condition at work.[25] Furthermore, little consideration is given to destigmatising poverty and other social determinants of mental illness and suicide.	Do not assume that the more we talk about and label people with mental illness, depression etc., the better it will be for people with those labels.
commit suicide The term 'commit suicide' is highly contentious in the suicide prevention/mental health sector. The word 'commit', when used in relation to suicide, has historically been conflated with criminality and the Christian religious idea of 'mortal sin'. It can cause complicated feelings of judgement, shame, and guilt to family members. There have also been difficulties with life insurance claims being denied. Although both these issues have been resolved to some extent, many people still believe it is inappropriate to use the word 'commit'.	If you prefer not to use the word 'commit' when discussing suicide, alternative terms include: 'died by suicide', 'ended his/her life', 'took his/her own life'.

4
Risk factors and protective factors

Suicide prevention activity should be informed by known risk factors and protective factors. There are many known risk factors associated with stress that can contribute to suicide. It is important for effective suicide prevention that we design and target prevention activities according to the prevalence and strength of the risk factors in different demographic groups.

Risk and protective factors for suicide and suicidality act at multiple levels. Consequently, responses to these factors need to be multi-layered and multi-sectoral. Health, education, welfare, housing, legal, financial, and transport sectors are all crucially important and need to be strategically considered in suicide prevention policy and programs. It is important that key agencies outside health/mental health are actively involved in suicide prevention.

Table 4. Risk factors and protective factors

Term	Explanation
adverse life events	Nearly all suicides appear to be associated with adverse (negative) life events within one year of death, often concentrated in the last few months prior to death.[37]
	The international literature on risk factors for suicide consistently identifies a range of adverse life events and stressful challenges associated with suicide. Precipitating events have been found in up to 96% of suicides, with studies showing that social factors play a key role in suicide risk.[38] Relevant adverse life events include unemployment, relationship breakdown, collapse of a business, prolonged drought in farming communities, and serious health problems and illness or death of family members. Often there is no single event but rather the accumulation of a series of adverse life events, described in published research as 'pathways to despair'.[39]
at-risk	In general, 'at-risk' people are individuals and groups who have higher rates of suicide and suicidality compared with the general population.
	Identifying people at-risk can play an important role in helping focus preventive activities.
risk factors	Risk factors are events or circumstances that negatively impact on a person's life and potentially increase the likelihood of suicide and self-harm.
	Key risk factors for suicide include social determinants such as unemployment, financial difficulties and homelessness, as well as high-intensity psychological difficulties, mental disorders, prior suicide attempts, alcohol and other drug misuse, serious health challenges, child abuse and other adverse childhood experiences (ACEs), psychological trauma, grief, separation and divorce, and the experience of powerlessness. Risk factors vary in relation to age, gender, and other intersecting social and cultural factors. However, the evidence suggests that in many cases, perhaps the majority of cases, multiple risk factors at multiple levels combine to elevate psychological distress to intolerable levels. Several risk factors may be influential at multiple levels and may overlap.[40]

Risk factors and protective factors

Term	Explanation
proximal risk factors	Proximal risk factors are events or circumstances that have a more direct and immediate influence on a person's level of psychological distress.
	Proximal risk factors may exacerbate existing life challenges. They include adverse life events/circumstances such as the failure of a person's business, farm repossession, job loss, relationship breakdown, and serious health issues.[41] They also include access to means of suicide (e.g. guns or drugs).
distal risk factors	Distal risk factors are historical and contextual factors that may increase the risk of suicide.
	Examples of distal risk factors include child abuse and other ACEs, sustained poverty, social isolation, poor social service support, and traumatic experiences of military personnel and veterans.[42]
protective factors	Protective factors are aspects of a person's life/circumstances that reduce the risk of suicide.
	Protective factors may be present in all aspects of a person's life, throughout the lifespan. Examples of key protective factors for people in distress include interpersonal and social support of family, friends, and/or work colleagues, and constructive help-seeking. Work can be a protective factor, above and beyond the financial benefits, providing social interaction/support, meaningful activity, and engendering self-esteem. For young people, a good school experience and positive peer and adult relationships are protective.[43]
	Other protective factors include policies and practices that restrict the means of suicide.[44]
	Effective, humane institutional and service/agency support is also protective, not only for suicide and self-harm prevention, but also to reduce the risk of other adverse outcomes such as unemployment, homelessness, and family breakdown.
	At the broader social level, protective factors need to be articulated and enshrined in social policies that address the social determinants of health and wellbeing.
	Protective factors are related to resilience, and have both individual and social dimensions. People can be more resilient in the face of adversity where there are good social support structures in place.

Language Matters

Term	Explanation
social determinants (SDH) (SDOH) (SDOMH)	Social determinants of health are social, economic, and material factors, including income, employment status, working conditions, education, housing, food security, transport, and social inclusion/(non)discrimination, all of which profoundly affect both physical and mental health. Social determinants are an appropriate focus for population-level mental health promotion. The acronyms 'SDOH' and 'SDH' are often used for social determinants of health. We use 'SDOMH' for social determinants of mental health. The Situational Approach to suicide prevention and mental health has much in common with a SDOMH perspective at a population level, but it is more directly applicable at an individual/clinical level.
structural determinants	Structural determinants are root causes of health disparities, including political/economic/social policies and regulatory and administrative processes, that affect income, working conditions, housing, and education, etc. Structural determinants overlap with social determinants, but the term more specifically refers to political and economic factors. For example, unemployment is a social determinant, whereas government employment policy is a structural determinant. HR policy can be considered as a more proximal structural determinant. It is strongly influenced by government policy and economic trends, but it is also influenced by factors such as industry characteristics/demands (e.g. rostering/shift-work) and specific workplace cultures (e.g., white-collar, blue-collar, hospitality industry). Personal attitudes can also shape HR policy, particularly in small organisations.
biopsychosocial factors	Biopsychosocial factors are a broad range of factors that potentially affect health and wellbeing. An individual's health and wellbeing are influenced by their biology, environmental factors, and psychological and social factors. The idea of interacting systems at both the individual and social level is a core concept of the biopsychosocial model.[45] Even intense 'inner' psychological distress should be seen as part of a broader set of influences. Resolution of this distress can often only be achieved by acknowledging and working with these interactive factors, including those outside the individual's influence or control. Unfortunately, the term 'biopsychosocial' is often inappropriately applied to strongly biological perspectives that merely pay lip-service to social factors and social needs.[46]

5

The spectrum of suicide prevention activity

Currently, suicide prevention initiatives occur across a broad spectrum of activity representing two broadly different orientations and approaches (Figure 1). The different models can generally be understood as:

(1) broadscale, population-wide strategies
(2) more targeted strategies such as support for individuals who are acutely distressed and at-risk, and follow-up support for people bereaved by suicide and for people who have non-fatally self-harmed.

Figure 1. The suicide prevention spectrum

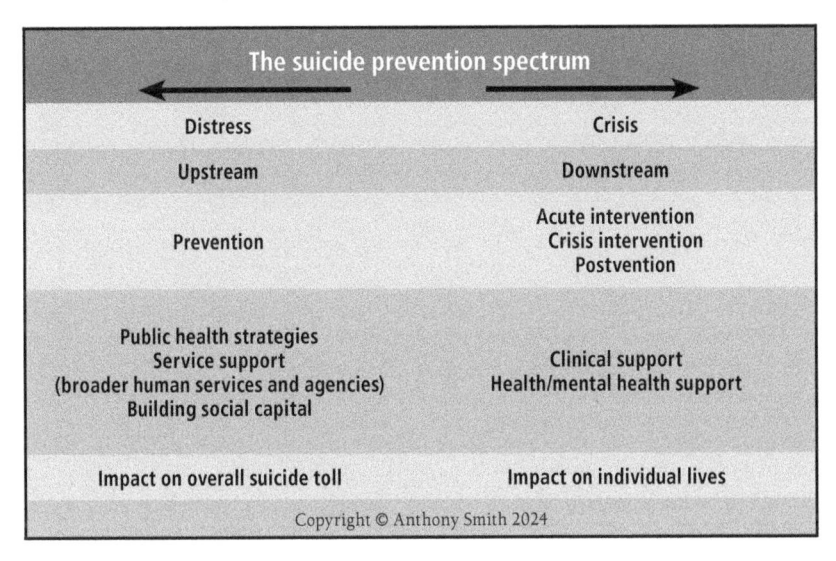

Distress	Crisis
Upstream	Downstream
Prevention	Acute intervention Crisis intervention Postvention
Public health strategies Service support (broader human services and agencies) Building social capital	Clinical support Health/mental health support
Impact on overall suicide toll	Impact on individual lives

Copyright © Anthony Smith 2024

There are different levels of prevention. Much of the current approach to suicide prevention sits within the downstream, acute level of intervention. Although important in responding to people identified as being at elevated risk of suicide, this level of intervention fails to alter the trajectory of escalating risk for many people who go on to kill themselves. Such interventions cannot be expected to reduce the overall toll of suicide. The limited impact of downstream interventions on the suicide toll is further compounded by ineffectual upstream interventions that are influenced by mental illness ideology, for example the promotion of depression screening, despite evidence that it is ineffective and may even be harmful.[47]

Health and human service agency responses to suicide in Australia are generally referred to with the generic term 'suicide prevention'. However, much of the work done in this field, although important, is not so much preventive as a reactive response to the tragedy of suicide. Although reactive interventions can have an important preventive role – such as providing follow-up support for people personally affected by suicide – they have limited preventive impact at the population level.[48]

Effective suicide prevention requires that all levels of intervention be evidence-based and subjected to rigorous evaluation.[49] Unfortunately, there is often a sort of exceptionalism operating in suicide prevention and management, whereby evidence of effectiveness and safety is not considered necessary for interventions to be implemented and maintained.[50] For example, treatment is regarded as necessary and urgent, even if it is not evidence-based. There is often pressure to 'do *something*', even if there is no evidence to support the chosen intervention.

The spectrum of suicide prevention activity

Table 5. Suicide prevention levels and strategies

Term	Explanation
upstream prevention	Upstream prevention addresses financial, environmental, industrial and economic structures and conditions – social/structural determinants – that may impact negatively on the wellbeing of many people in the overall population or in population subgroups.
	Key factors in suicide such as unemployment, financial difficulties, and housing insecurity often cause intense distress. Appropriate population-level interventions to support people experiencing these challenges should primarily focus on activity outside the health/mental health sector, such as job-creation, re-employment support, housing affordability policies, and financial support programs.
	Effective upstream prevention activity, focusing on populations/subgroups, not individuals, is required to reduce the overall toll of suicide. To be effective, upstream prevention activity should address fundamental social and economic structures that can enable improved social support and general protective factors across the total population. Ultimately, what is needed are changes at a political level to reduce disadvantage and inequality.
	Common upstream prevention activities in the health/welfare sector include community outreach services, public awareness campaigns, and community education.
	Health professionals can also take an advocacy role in lobbying governments to develop population-level initiatives in relevant departments such as housing, employment, welfare, and finance.[51]
downstream prevention	Downstream prevention refers to activity that is generally limited to dealing directly with individuals who have been identified as at-risk of suicide, and/or ongoing postvention support (e.g. counselling/psychotherapy) for family and friends affected by suicide and suicidality.
	Although downstream prevention is vitally important in caring for highly distressed individuals, it cannot play a major role in reducing the overall toll of suicide. This is in large part because many people who die by suicide do not have meaningful engagement, if any engagement at all, with health/support services prior to their death.

Language Matters

Term	Explanation
universal prevention strategies[52]	Universal prevention strategies address an entire population (e.g. all residents of a state or country) or cohort (e.g. all primary school students), not just people considered to be at risk. Universal prevention strategies include programs such as public education campaigns, means restriction, education programs for the media on reporting practices related to suicide, and crisis response plans.
selective prevention strategies	Selective prevention strategies address subsets of the total population, focusing on at-risk groups who have a greater probability of becoming suicidal. This level of prevention includes screening programs and training for frontline caregivers and peer support workers and is designed to prevent the onset and escalation of suicidal behaviours among specific subpopulations.
indicated prevention strategies	Indicated strategies address high-risk individuals and groups within the population – people experiencing personal crises and/or showing signs of high-intensity psychological distress, who may be at high risk of suicide. Indicated strategies are generally delivered by services and organisations such as crisis helplines, referral services, and survivor postvention services.[53]
public health interventions	Public health interventions are population-wide approaches by the health sector, often in collaboration with other sectors, including housing, employment, education and transport. Public health interventions in suicide prevention are generally universal prevention strategies, e.g. barriers on the sides of bridges, to prevent anyone climbing over and jumping off (or risking falling off). Appropriate public health activity built on good research and planning represents an important opportunity to effectively address the suicide toll. However, public health activity in the mental health/suicide prevention sector (and the health sector more broadly) has tended to reflect a narrow medicalised approach: and where there have been attempts to advocate to broaden the focus to include social determinants such as poverty and housing, there has generally not been the political will to enact this in any substantial way.[54]
acute clinical intervention	Acute intervention refers to engagement by health/welfare workers with individuals who are so highly psychologically distressed that they may be at risk of self-harm or suicide. Acute intervention is important at the individual level, but it has limited preventive impact at the population level.[55]

The spectrum of suicide prevention activity

Term	Explanation
crisis intervention	Like acute intervention, crisis intervention refers to engaging directly with individuals who may be at high risk of self-harm or suicide.
	Ideally, crisis interventions would occur in broader settings than just the medical/mental health domain, and would include all relevant government agencies (such as housing and employment support) as well as not-for-profit and community care organisations.
suicide postvention	Suicide postvention generally refers to support for people who have been affected by a suicide death, but it can also include support for people who have attempted suicide, and their family and friends.[56]
	Grief counselling and support is vitally important for family and friends, who may be at increased risk of suicide themselves, because of their responses to the suicide (e.g. grief and/or guilt). However, like any other later intervention, postvention is limited in its scope of prevention, because it generally targets only people who have been identified by health/support services as being at-risk through their connection to individual suicide deaths or suicide attempts.

6
Understanding key concepts about research and practice

The effectiveness of research and practice in the mental health/suicide prevention sector has sometimes been hindered by misunderstandings of key concepts and inappropriate use of terminology. It is important for effective work in this sector that key concepts are properly understood and the corresponding terminology is used appropriately and consistently.

Understanding key concepts about research and practice

Table 6. Clarification of some key terms and concepts about research and practice

Term/concept	Clarification
rates versus numbers	Both population rates and actual/absolute numbers of suicide deaths are important for consideration of appropriate suicide prevention activity. However, either considered alone without reference to the other can give a distorted representation of suicide deaths.
	Rates of suicide are generally measured as deaths per 100,000 of a population group.[57] However, although this facilitates comparisons between different groups, it can give rise to a skewed representation when working with relatively small populations, such as in rural areas in Australia. High rates in a small population may justify specific targeted interventions, but this may not lead to a reduction in the overall toll if larger populations with larger numbers (but lower rates) of suicide deaths are not properly targeted as well.
	Absolute numbers are the total numbers of deaths in a defined area or group in a specified time period. For larger population areas or groups, relatively large numbers of suicide deaths in a specified time period may be reported/expressed as relatively lower rates and consequently may not receive the attention they warrant.
gender specificity in suicide prevention	The suicide/self-harm spectrum is strongly gender-specific. Although there is some overlap, the large majority (about 75%) of suicide deaths occur in males, but most recorded incidents of non-fatal self-harm occur in females.[58] Developing effective preventive activity on this suicide/self-harm spectrum requires clearly defined, evidence-based gender-specific activity on a scale proportionate to the risk level of the target group.
rural versus metropolitan suicide rates	In general, rural rates of suicide are higher than rates in metropolitan areas, and appropriate preventive activity is required to address this. However, the majority of Australian suicide deaths occur in city-dwelling adults.[59] Sydney, Melbourne, Brisbane, Adelaide and Perth together account for over half (54.18%) of all suicide deaths in Australia.
	Although rural rates of suicide are generally higher than metropolitan rates, this is a potentially misleading generalisation: rates vary enormously if measured by locality (for example, local government areas or federal electorates) in both rural and metropolitan areas.[60] Some metropolitan areas have both higher rates of suicide than many rural areas and considerably higher numbers of suicide deaths than many rural areas. Suicide rates tend to be higher in socially and economically disadvantaged areas, both metropolitan and rural.[61]

Language Matters

Term/concept	Clarification
groups with high rates of suicide	As well as high rates of suicide in some rural areas and socially and economically disadvantaged metropolitan areas, there are high rates among other groups, including among Aboriginal people, with very high rates among young Aboriginal males.[62]
	There are disproportionately high rates of suicide (and attempted suicide) among unemployed people. The majority of all suicide deaths occur in people who are not employed, and there are also high rates of suicide among mature-age men and unemployed people (both male and female).[63] Suicide deaths among people who are not employed account for at least 55% of all suicide deaths of people of working age. For women of working age, there is a particularly high proportion of suicide deaths among those who are not employed – 68.2%.
youth suicide	When youth suicide is discussed, 'youth' can refer to various age-groups, and people often equate 'youth' with 'teenage'.
	It is important to distinguish between the 15–19-year-old age-group and the 15–24-year-old age-group, because there are much larger numbers of suicide deaths in 20–24-year-olds than in 15–19-year-olds (older teenagers).[64] Adding the two age-groups together significantly inflates the 'youth' numbers. These inflated figures are then used to argue for program and research funding that largely targets teenagers, while very little suicide prevention activity targets the 20–24 age-group.
data collection, analysis, and reporting	Rigorous data gathering and analysis and unbiased reporting of evidence are vital for informing effective suicide prevention. Evidence that is viewed from a limited/biased perspective, particularly the unhelpful presumption that suicide is usually caused by mental disorders, disregarding situational factors, is inadequate for suicide research.
	The Australian Bureau of Statistics (ABS) publishes data on causes of death, including suicide. However, the risk factors for suicide included in ABS statistics are dominated by diagnostic categories such as mental disorders and substance abuse disorders,[65] while little attention has been paid to important social determinants such as unemployment and housing difficulties.[66]

Understanding key concepts about research and practice

Term/concept	Clarification
appropriate research methodology	Effective suicide prevention requires good research. It should be rigorously evidence-based, with strong ethical underpinnings. Overall, there should be an appropriate balance between quantitative research and qualitative research (including lived experience). There needs to be a major focus on social/structural determinants of health/mental health. However, there is strong criticism of current approaches to suicide prevention research. Knox (2014) expressed this well: *To date, research has been insufficient to explain why men, especially during middle age, are particularly vulnerable to taking their own lives. The shortcomings of prior studies include lack of longitudinal follow-up, failure to measure such factors as social integration and dimensional indicators of stress, overreliance on categorical measures of psychopathology, and a focus on proxy outcomes instead of death by suicide.*[67] Note: 'Proxy outcomes' include measures of things like attempted suicide, depressive symptom severity, suicidality, loneliness, and indicators of psychopathology.[68] Suicide prevention research tends to be dominated by a focus on mental illness, particularly depression, and assumptions such as the importance of screening for mental disorders and providing clinical treatment. Although people who are at risk of suicide and who have already come to the attention of health services are one important focus of research, clinical research offers little opportunity for guidance in moving towards more effective population-wide prevention.

Term/concept	Clarification
evidence and evidence base	Research and practice that is evidence-based has robust methodology and a sound rationale for claims of effectiveness.
	It is vital that suicide prevention activities are underpinned by robust evidence. For example, because there are many different target groups requiring different approaches, properly defining target groups, and developing appropriate evidence-based prevention strategies, is crucial.[69]
	Much of the current approach to suicide prevention is at odds with much of the available evidence, and disregards contrary evidence that doesn't suit organisational or business agendas. It is often too generic and reductionist to be effective. It lacks crucial gender differentiation, applies a narrow clinical lens, and tends to ignore robust research highlighting important social determinants of suicide, such as unemployment.[70]
	The term 'evidence-based' is often misused and can sometimes serve to endorse and reinforce aspects of the current approach within the mental health/suicide prevention sector.[71]
biomedical model	The biomedical approach interprets patterns of behaviour and psychological distress as symptomatic of mental disorders or illnesses. People are viewed simply as patients to be diagnosed and treated by medical means, often potentially harmful antidepressant drugs.[72]
	The biomedical model of mental health has borrowed heavily from the general medical sector. It presumes pathology at the biological level of individuals as the basis of psychological/emotional problems. This ideology has given rise to widespread acceptance of 'chemical imbalances' as explaining distress and requiring drug treatment, when evidence clearly disproves any such causal explanation.[73]
	This individualised approach tends to ignore social, contextual/situational factors and influences, reinforcing the pathologising and medicalising of common human experiences.

Understanding key concepts about research and practice

Term/concept	Clarification
mental health ideology	The term 'ideology' refers to systematically related beliefs and assumptions that form the basis of a more-or-less coherent perspective. Mental health ideology refers to the broader set of beliefs justifying an over-medicalised approach to distress and other common human behaviours. The dominant narrative about mental health is founded on the biomedical model, which is rarely questioned. Using clinical terminology such as 'symptom', 'illness', and 'treatment' in relation to people in distress helps to establish and maintain mental illness ideology. It also helps to legitimise the over-medicalised approach, and influences people to accept it as valid and authoritative. Although the term 'mental health ideology' may be confrontational to some people, understanding the influence of ideology is important to help counter the prevailing biomedical narrative.
medicalisation	A key part of the biomedical model is the concept of medicalisation. To medicalise is to reduce and simplify issues of personal health and wellbeing to medical diagnoses, often presuming the need for medical treatment.[74] For suicide prevention, this refers to the process of reducing complex issues of psychological or emotional distress, regardless of the causes of that distress, to medical diagnoses such as depression or anxiety disorder. This is usually followed by treatment, commonly including prescription of potentially harmful pharmaceuticals such as antidepressants or antipsychotics (for depression and anxiety disorders) and amphetamine derivatives (for children's behavioural issues).[75] Other typical medicalisation processes include consulting with a GP who diagnoses a mental disorder and develops a Mental Health Treatment Plan,[76] without properly considering life circumstances and alternative ways of addressing stressors. This is not to suggest that appropriate medical intervention is never warranted, but such intervention should always be integrated with a broader contextual, situational approach to support.
pathologisation	Pathologisation is a similar process to medicalisation – interpreting and describing common human experiences as medical abnormalities, disorders or illnesses. This is all too common in the suicide prevention sector, where the symptoms of stress, particularly strong psychological distress, are presumed to be evidence of a mental disorder in the individual rather than reflecting their relationships and life circumstances.

Language Matters

Term/concept	Clarification
workplace mental health (WMH)	Workplace mental health (WMH) has become a major workplace issue. However, WMH usually has a medicalised and individualised orientation, focusing more on individuals identified and diagnosed as having mental health problems than on promotion of wellbeing and prevention of problems.
	An individualistic approach is sometimes appropriate, for example in management of worker compensation claims, where a person-centred focus can be helpful. However, it should not dominate WMH practice, because it deflects attention from workplace conditions that may jeopardise the mental health of many workers.
	Paradoxically, the medicalisation that dominates WMH may also be detrimental to workers and, furthermore, to employers and to the sustainability of the superannuation/life insurance industries.[77]
	There is international concern about increasing numbers of workers on sickness and disability benefits, with diagnoses of mental disorders disproportionately increasing.[78] In Australia, work-related mental health conditions are now the second most common cause of workers' compensation claims.[79]
	Regardless of the factors causing workplace stress or trauma, many WMH policies and practices for dealing with worker distress give workers little option but to accept a medicalised pathway and the diagnosis of a mental disorder if they wish to receive ongoing workplace accommodations and/or financial support.[80]
	WMH insurance claims are made to support distressed workers. However, WMH literature generally uses medicalised language and promotes a medicalised approach to 'mental health conditions'. For example, the TAL (a leading Australian life insurance company) 'Understanding mental health' webpage states:
	Mental health conditions are diagnosed based on a history of symptoms reported to and observed by a mental health professional[81]
	Despite the efforts and enormous funding to destigmatise mental illness, and the encouragement and messaging for people to 'talk to someone about your mental health', recent data shows that more than half (53%) of Australian workers would hide a mental or physical health condition they had so that they would not be judged or discriminated against.[82] The lack of effectiveness of destigmatisation efforts has led one high-profile leader in the mental health arena to openly recommend that people not disclose their mental health issues to employers.[83]

Understanding key concepts about research and practice

Term/concept	Clarification
workplace mental health training	Workplace mental health training has become a lucrative business[84] and most employers are obliged to provide such training. However, much of the training is built around diagnostic labels and other clinical terminology.[85] Although there is now some acknowledgement in WMH training (and HR policy more broadly) of difficult workplace conditions (e.g. long hours, shift-work, lack of job control) and stressful workplace events (e.g. harassment, bullying, violence and stigmatisation of mental health problems), there is still very little attention given to social determinants such as poverty and housing insecurity. More appropriate WMH training would include a focus on both work-related factors and personal/domestic factors that can affect workers' mental health. It would emphasise the importance of consideration of the work situation of workers, particularly factors that might impact stress levels, such as zero-hour contracts or other insecure working conditions. Appropriate WMH training would highlight the responsibility of workplace management to investigate causes of distress, and to implement strategies to reduce stressors within the workplace. Additionally, it would present and promote options for appropriate interventions and supportive strategies, both reactive and proactive. More appropriate training would help to minimise pathologising language and help reduce the number of people who are directed to GPs for diagnoses of mental disorders. WMH training should also consider the human costs of over-medicalisation, including overdiagnosis of mental disorders and over-prescribing of antidepressants and other psychotropic drugs. International research confirms that stigmatisation of mental health problems is prevalent in the workplace and impacts upon workers and work conditions and processes such as employment/reemployment.[86] Furthermore, over-medicalisation has substantial economic costs, particularly related to long-term sick leave and permanent disability support pensions.[87]

Language Matters

Term/concept	Clarification
the 'talk to someone' message	The 'talk to someone' message as a preventive strategy is popular and widespread, and has attracted substantial support in mental health campaigns.[88] Talking to someone is particularly advocated in relation to men, because they are less likely to seek help, both formal and informal.[89] However, the evidence for the value of talking to someone as a population-wide preventive activity is questionable. The occasional anecdotal story of a distressed person who talked to someone and received help, although a favourite with the media, does not constitute evidence of its effectiveness. Published research paints a different picture, with recent research showing that this sort of strategy leads a significant proportion of people (especially men) onto a very problematic and potentially tragic pathway.[90] *Rather than a focus on 'talk' as a response to suicide among men, suicide prevention initiatives might instead seek to engage more broadly with economic and housing security, access to non-stigmatizing welfare/disability support, robust programs promoting gender equality, easy access to well-resourced community-based services in relation to mental health and substance use.*[91] There are important questions to ask about the 'talk to someone' message. Who should people speak with if they are in crisis? What are the appropriate skills for supportive engagement of people whose distress is clearly related to adverse life events? Research has shown that this particular approach may be particularly unhelpful for some men: *It may be the case that common suicide prevention strategies, such as encouraging greater use of mental health services by men and focusing on raising awareness of links between mental illness and suicide, are unlikely to lead to effective interventions for such individuals.*[92]

Acknowledgements

The *Language Matters* guide is a companion to the book *Default Depression – How we now interpret distress as mental illness.*

Acknowledgements

We acknowledge John Ashfield PhD for his important contribution in the development of new terms in the key Situational Approach documents. Julia Beaven, Senior Editor at Wakefield Press, edited the section (Appendix D) in the *Default Depression* book which forms the basis of this document. The late Dr John Walsh also made valuable contributions. Other sources have been acknowledged as references.

Contributions from people with lived experience

There have been significant contributions and feedback made to the development of *Default Depression* and *Language Matters* by a number of people with lived experience. Most recently LELAN (SA Lived Experience Leadership & Advocacy Network) offered suggestions about terminology relevant to Table 5.

> *Suggested citation:* Smith A., Raven M. (2024). *Language Matters: Appropriate Language Guide for Supporting People in Distress* (Version 1). Wakefield Press.

Notes

1 Ashfield J., Macdonald J. & Smith A. (2017) Situational Approach to Suicide Prevention: Why we need a paradigm shift for effective suicide prevention. https://doi.org/10.25155/2017/150417; Ashfield J., Macdonald J., Francis A. & Smith A. (2017) A 'Situational Approach' to Mental Health Literacy in Australia: Redefining mental health literacy to empower communities for preventative mental health, https://doi.org/10.25155/2017/150517. 14

2 Ashfield J., Macdonald J., Francis A. & Smith A. (2017) A 'Situational Approach' to Mental Health Literacy in Australia: Redefining mental health literacy to empower communities for preventative mental health, https://doi.org/10.25155/2017/150517. 14

3 Smith P., Jostmann N.B., Galinsky A.D., & van Dijk W.W. (2008) Lacking power impairs executive functions. *Psychological Science, 19*(5), 441–447. doi:10.1111/j.1467-9280.2008.02107.x

4 Ashfield J., Macdonald J. & Smith A. (2017) Situational Approach to Suicide Prevention: Why we need a paradigm shift for effective suicide prevention. https://doi.org/10.25155/2017/150417: Hockey M., Rocks T., Ruusunen A., Jacka F., Huang W., Liao B., Aune D., Wang Y., Nie J. & O'Neil A. (2021) Psychological distress as a risk factor for all-cause, chronic disease and suicide-specific mortality: a prospective analysis using data from the National Health Interview Survey. *Social Psychiatry and Psychiatric Epidemiology, 57*(3). 541–552

5 Tang S., Reily N.M., Arena A.F., Batterham P.J., Calear A.L., Carter G.L., Mackinnon A.J. & Christensen H. (2022) People who die by suicide without receiving mental health services: A systematic review. *Frontiers in Public Health*, 9. doi:10.3389/fpubh.2021.736948

6 Tang S., Reily N.M., Arena A.F., Batterham P.J., Calear A.L., Carter G.L., Mackinnon A.J. & Christensen H. (2022) People who die by suicide

Notes

without receiving mental health services: A systematic review. *Frontiers in Public Health*, 9. doi:10.3389/fpubh.2021.736948; McPhedran S. & De Leo D. (2013) Miseries suffered, unvoiced, unknown? Communication of suicidal intent by men in "rural" Queensland, Australia. *Suicide and Life-Threatening Behavior*: 5, https://doi.org/10.1111/sltb.12041; Foster T. (2011) Adverse Life Events Proximal to Adult Suicide: A Synthesis of Findings from Psychological Autopsy Studies, Archives of Suicide Research 15, 1: 1–15, doi: 10.1080/13811118.2011.540213

7 Saar E. & Burgess T. (2016) Intentional Self-Harm Fatalities in Australia 2001–2013. Data Report DR16-16. National Coronial Information System. http://malesuicidepreventionaustralia.com.au/wp-content/uploads/2017/01/NCIS-Report-2016_FINAL.pdf. Table 1: Intentional Self-Harm Fatalities in Australia by Employment Status and Age Range

8 McPhedran S. & De Leo D. (2013) Miseries suffered, unvoiced, unknown? Communication of suicidal intent by men in "rural" Queensland, Australia, *Suicide and Life-Threatening Behavior*. The American Association of Suicidology DOI: 10.1111/sltb.12041; Laanani M., Imbaud C., Tuppin P., Poulalhon C., Jollant F., Coste J. & Rey G. (2020) Contacts with health services during the year prior to suicide death and prevalent conditions a nationwide study. *Journal of Affective Disorders*, 274, 174–182. doi:10.1016/j.jad.2020.05.071; Mughal F. Bojanić L., Rodway C., Graney J., Ibrahim S., Quinlivan L., Steeg S., Tham S.G., Turnbull P., Appleby L., Webb R.T., & Kapur N. (2023) Recent GP consultation before death by suicide in middle-aged males: A national consecutive case series study, *British Journal of General Practice*, 73(732). doi:10.3399/bjgp.2022.0589; Pearson A., Saini P., Da Cruz D., Miles C., While D., Swinson N., Williams A., Shaw J., Appleby L., Kapur N. (2009) Primary care contact prior to suicide in individuals with mental illness. *British Journal of General Practice*. 59(568):825–32. doi:10.3399/bjgp09X472881

9 Staiger T., Maja S., Mueller-Stierlin A.S., Kilian R., Beschoner P., Gündel H., Becker T., Frasch K., Panzirsch M., Schmauß M. & Krumm S. (2020) Masculinity and help-seeking among men with depression: A qualitative study. *Frontiers in Psychiatry*, 11. doi:10.3389/fpsyt.2020.599039

10 Vickery A. (2021) Men's Help-Seeking for Distress: Navigating Varied Pathways and Practices. *Frontiers in Sociology*. 26;6:724843. doi: 10.3389/fsoc.2021.724843

11 Seidler Z. (2019) We tell men to open up more. But are we ready to listen?, *Age*, 18 October https://www.theage.com.au/lifestyle/life-and-relationships/we-tell-men-to-open-up-more-but-are-we-ready-to-listen-20191017-p531mg.html

12 Indigenous Mental Health & Suicide Prevention Clearinghouse. (2022) Social & emotional wellbeing. Australian Institute of Health and Welfare. https://www.indigenousmhspc.gov.au/

13 Australian Bureau of Statistics. (2023) National Study of Mental Health and Wellbeing. Summary statistics on key mental health issues including national and state and territory estimates of prevalence of mental disorders, Reference period 2020-2022. https://www.abs.gov.au/statistics/health/mental-health/national-study-mental-health-and-wellbeing/2020-2022#use-of-services

14 Safe Work Australia & Superfriend (2017/2021) Taking Action: A best practice framework for the management of psychological claims in the Australian workers' compensation sector. https://www.safeworkaustralia.gov.au/doc/taking-action-best-practice-framework-management-psychological-claims-australian-workers-compensation-sector (p. 66)

15 Safe Work Australia & Superfriend (2017/2021) Taking Action: A best practice framework for the management of psychological claims in the Australian workers' compensation sector. https://www.safeworkaustralia.gov.au/doc/taking-action-best-practice-framework-management-psychological-claims-australian-workers-compensation-sector

16 WorkSafe Victoria (2024) Mental injury support. https://www.worksafe.vic.gov.au/mental-injury-support

17 Safe Work Australia (2024) Psychosocial hazards. https://www.safeworkaustralia.gov.au/safety-topic/managing-health-and-safety/mental-health/psychosocial-hazards

18 Safe Work Australia & Superfriend (2017/2021) Taking Action: A best practice framework for the management of psychological claims in the Australian workers' compensation sector. https://www.safeworkaustralia.gov.au/doc/taking-action-best-practice-framework-management-psychological-claims-australian-workers-compensation-sector; Black Dog Institute (2024). How to manage psychosocial hazards in the workplace https://www.blackdoginstitute.org.au/news/how-to-manage-psychosocial-hazards-in-your-workplace' WorkSafe Victoria (2024) Mental injury support. https://www.worksafe.vic.gov.au/mental-injury-support

19 Safe Work Australia (2022) Managing psychosocial hazards at work: Code of Practice (p. 5) https://www.safeworkaustralia.gov.au/sites/default/files/2022-08/model_code_of_practice_-managing_psychosocial_hazards_at_work_25082022_0.pdf

20 Jorm A.F., Korten A.E., Jacomb P.A., Christensen H., Rodgers B., Pollitt P. et al. (1997) "Mental health literacy": a survey of the public's ability to recognise mental disorders and their beliefs about the effectiveness

Notes

of treatment. *Med J Aust.* 166(4):182–186. doi:10.5694/j.1326-5377.1997.tb140071.x

21 Bjornsen H.N., Eilertsen M-E.B., Ringdal R., Espnes G.A. & Moksnes U.K. (2017) Positive mental health literacy: development and validation of a measure among Norwegian adolescents *BMC Public Health* 17, 717 (2017). https://doi.org/10.1186/s12889-017-4733-6

22 Foulkes L. & Andrews J.L. (2023) Are mental health awareness efforts contributing to the rise in reported mental health problems? A call to test the prevalence inflation hypothesis. *New Ideas in Psychology*, 69, 101010. doi:10.1016/j.newideapsych.2023.101010

23 Smith A., (2021) Focus on individual wellbeing doesn't help. *Guardian*, 8 May https://www.theguardian.com/society/2021/may/08/the-self-help-cult-of-resilience-teaches-australians-nothing; Donoghue, M. (2021) Resilience, discipline and financialisation in the UK's liberal welfare state. *New Political Economy*. https://www.tandfonline.com/doi/full/10.1080/13563467.2021.1994538 (8 November 2021); Hickman P. (2017) A Flawed Construct? Understanding and Unpicking the Concept of Resilience in the Context of Economic Hardship. *Social Policy and Society* 17(3), 409–424

24 Hodges E., Leditschke A. & Solonsch L. (2023) The Lived Experience Governance Framework: Centring People, Identity and Human Rights for the Benefit of All. https://nmhccf.org.au/our-work/discussion-papers/the-lived-experience-governance-framework-centring-people-identity-and-human-rights-for-the-benefit-of-all

25 Australian College of Applied Professions. (2021) Nationally Representative Survey of Australian Workers. https://www.acap.edu.au/wp-content/uploads/2021/12/Executive-Summary-ACAP-results-002-1.pdf

26 AIHW. (2023) Suicide & self-harm monitoring Australian Government. https://www.aihw.gov.au/suicide-self-harm-monitoring/data/deaths-by-suicide-in-australia/prevalence-estimates-of-suicidal-behaviours

27 Turecki G. & Brent D.A. (2015) Suicide and suicidal behaviour. *Lancet 387*, 10024, 1227–1239. doi:10.1016/S0140-6736(15)00234-2

28 Bostwick M.J., Pabbati C., Geske J.R. & McKean A.J. (2016) Suicide attempt as a risk factor for completed suicide: Even more lethal than we knew. *American Journal of Psychiatry*, 173(11), 1094–1100. doi:10.1176/appi.ajp.2016.15070854

29 Raven M., Smith A., & Jureidini J. (2017) Suicide and Self-Harm in Australia: Conceptual Map. (Paper presented at the Royal Australian and New Zealand College of Psychiatrists Congress, Adelaide, South Australia, 30 April – 4 May 2017), http://malesuicidepreventionaustralia.com.au/wp-content/uploads/2017/05/Suicide_and_Self_Harm_in_Australia.pdf

30 Beautrais A. (2001) Suicides and serious suicide attempts: two populations or one? *Psychological Medicine 31*, 5:837, doi:10.1017/s0033291701003889; Nock M.K., Borges G., Bromet E.J., Cha C.B., Kessler R.C. & Lee S. (2008). Suicide and suicidal behavior. *Epidemiologic Reviews 30*: 144, doi:10.1093/epirev/mxn002

31 Isometsä E.T. & Lönnqvist J.K. (1998) Suicide attempts preceding completed suicide. *British Journal of Psychiatry*, 173, 531–535. https://doi.org/10.1192/bjp.173.6.531; Bostwick J.M., Pabbati C., Geske J.R. & McKean A.J. (2016) Suicide attempt as a risk factor for completed suicide: Even more lethal than we knew. *American Journal of Psychiatry*, 173(11), 1094–1100. https://pubmed.ncbi.nlm.nih.gov/27523496/

32 Harrison J. & Henley G. (2014) Suicide and hospitalised self-harm in Australia: trends and analysis. Canberra: AIHW, https://www.aihw.gov.au/getmedia/b70c6e73-40dd-41ce-9aa4-b72b2a3dd152/18303.pdf; Hawton K., Rodham K., Evans E. & Weatherall R. (2002) Deliberate self-harm in adolescents: self report survey in schools in England, *BMJ* 325: 1207–1211, doi:10.1136/bmj.325.7374.120; Mental Health Foundation (2024) The Truth about Self-Harm. https://www.mentalhealth.org.uk/publications/truth-about-self-harm

33 Laye-Gindhu A. & Schonert-Reichl K.A. (2005) Nonsuicidal Self-Harm Among Community Adolescents: Understanding the "Whats" and "Whys" of Self-Harm. *Journal of Youth and Adolescence 34*, 5: 447–457, doi:10.1007/s10964-005-7262-z; Klonsky E.D. (2007) The functions of deliberate self-injury: A review of the evidence. *Clinical Psychological Review 27*, 2: 226–239, doi:10.1016/j.cpr.2006.08.002; Muehlenkamp J.J. (2005) Self-Injurious Behavior as a Separate Clinical Syndrome. *American Journal of Orthopsychiatry 75*, 2): 324–333, doi:10.1037/0002-9432.75.2.324

34 AIHW. Suicide & self-harm monitoring. (2024) https://www.aihw.gov.au/suicide-self-harm-monitoring/data/deaths-by-suicide-in-australia/prevalence-estimates-of-suicidal-behaviours; Hawton K., Bale L., Brand F., Townsend E., Ness J., Waters K., Clements C., Kapur N. & Geulayov G. (2020) Mortality in children and adolescents following presentation to hospital after non-fatal self-harm in the Multicentre Study of Self-harm: a prospective observational cohort study. *Lancet Child Adolesc Health*. 4(2):111–120. doi: 10.1016/S2352-4642(19)30373-6

35 Raven M., Smith A. & Jureidini J. (2017) Suicide and Self-Harm in Australia: Conceptual Map. (Paper presented at the Royal Australian and New Zealand College of Psychiatrists Congress, Adelaide, South Australia, 30 April – 4 May 2017), http://malesuicidepreventionaustralia.com.au/wp-content/uploads/2017/05/Suicide_and_Self_Harm_in_Australia.pdf

36 Uh S., Dalmaijer E.S., Siugzdaite R., Ford T.J. & Astle D.E. (2021) Two Pathways to Self-Harm in Adolescence. *Journal of the American Academy*

Notes

of Adolescent Psychiatry. 60(12):1491–1500. doi:10.1016/j.jaac.2021.03.010. Witt K., Milner A., Spittal M.J., Hetrick S., Robinson J., Pirkis J. & Carter G. (2018) Population attributable risk of factors associated with the repetition of self-harm behaviour in young people presenting to clinical services: a systematic review and meta-analysis. *European]Child and Adolescent Psychiatry 28*, 5–18. doi:10.1007/s00787-018-1111-6; Plener P.L., Schumacher, T.S., Munz L.M. & Groschwitz R.C. (2015) The longitudinal course of non-suicidal self-injury and deliberate self-harm: a systematic review of the literature. *Borderline Personality Disorder and Emotional Dysregulation.* 2:2. doi:10.1186/s40479-014-0024-3; Hawton K., Saunders K.E.A. & O'Connor R.C. (2012) Self-harm and suicide in adolescents. *Lancet, 379*(9834), 2373–2382. https://doi.org/10.1016/s0140-6736(12)60322-5

37 Foster T. (2011) Adverse Life Events Proximal to Adult Suicide: A Synthesis of Findings from Psychological Autopsy Studies. *Archives of Suicide Research 15*, 1 : 1–15, doi:10.1080/13811118.2011.540213

38 Almasi K., Belso, N., Kapur N., Webb R., Cooper J., Hadley S., Kerfoot M., Dunn G., Sotonyi P., Rihmer Z. & Appleby L. (2009) Risk factors for suicide in Hungary: a case-control study. *BMC Psychiatry 9*, 1 doi: 10.1186/1471-244x-9-45; Duberstein P., Conwell Y., Conner K.R., Eberly S., Evinger J.S. & Caine E.D. (2004) Poor social integration and suicide: fact or artefact? A case-control study. *Psychological Medicine 34*, 7: 1331–1337, doi:10.1017/s0033291704002600; De Leo D., Bille-Brahe U., Kerkhof A. & Schmidtke A. (eds), (2004) *Suicidal behaviour: Theories and research findings.* Ashland, Ohio: Hogrefe & Huber Publishers

39 Macdonald J.J., Smith, A., Gethin A., Sliwka G., Monaem A. & Powell K. (2016) Pathways to despair: a study of male suicide (aged 25–44). *Public Health Research* 4: 62–70, http://article.sapub.org/10.5923.j.phr.20140402.03.html

40 Public Health Association of Australia. (2018) Suicide Prevention Policy Position Statement. https://phaa.net.au/common/Uploaded%20files/SIG%20documents/Mental%20Health%20SIG/2021%20policy%20review%20-%2012-06%20-%20Suicide%20Prevention.pdf

41 Suicide Prevention Resource Center (2019) Topics and terms. https://sprc.org/topics-and-terms/

42 Seidler Z. (2019) We tell men to open up more. But are we ready to listen?' *Age*, 18 October 2019 https://www.theage.com.au/lifestyle/life-and-relationships/we-tell-men-to-open-up-more-but-are-we-ready-to-listen-20191017-p531mg.html

43 Butler N., Quigg Z., Bates R., Jones L., Ashworth E., Gowland S., Jones M. (2022) The Contributing Role of Family, School, and Peer Supportive Relationships in Protecting the Mental Wellbeing of Children

and Adolescents. *School Ment Health.* 14(3):776–788. doi:10.1007/s12310-022-09502-9

44 Hawton K. (2007) Restricting access to methods of suicide: Rationale and evaluation of this approach to suicide prevention. *Crisis: Journal of Crisis Intervention and Suicide Prevention.* 28(Supp 1). 4-9 https//doi.org/10.1027/0227-5910,28.S1.4; Yip P.S.F. Caine E., Yousuf S., Chang, S.S., Wu K.C. & Chen Y.Y. (2012) Means restriction for suicide prevention. *Lancet.* 379(9834):2393-9. doi:10.1016/S0140-6736(12)60521-2

45 Gask L. (2018) In defence of the biopsychosocial model. *Lancet Psychiatry* 5, 7: 548, doi:10.1016/s2215-0366(18)30165-2; Papadimitriou G.N. (2017) The "Biopsychosocial Model": 40 years of application in Psychiatry. *Psychiatriki* 282: 107–110, doi:10.22365/jpsych.2017.282.107; Thorpe R.J. & Halides P.N. (2016) Biopsychosocial Determinants of the Health of Boys and Men Across the Lifespan. *Behavioral Medicine* 42, 3: 129–131, doi:10.1080/08964289.2016.1191231; McInerney S.J. (2002) What is a good doctor and how can we make one? *BMJ 324* doi:10.1136/bmj.324.7353.1537/a; Deacon B.J. (2012) The biomedical model of mental disorder: A critical analysis of its validity, utility, and effects on psychotherapy research, *Clinical Psychology Review,* 33(7), 846–861. doi:10.1016/j.cpr.2012.09.007

46 Read J. (2005) The bio-bio-bio model of madness. *Psychologist.* 18(10), 596–597. https://www.bps.org.uk/psychologist/bio-bio-bio-model-madness

47 Cosgrove L., Karter J.M., Vaswani A. & Thombs B.D. (2018) Unexamined assumptions and unintended consequences of routine screening for depression. *Journal of Psychosomatic Research,* 109, 9–11. https://doi.org/10.1016/j.jpsychores.2018.03.007; Löwe B., Scherer M., Braunschneider L.E., Marx G., Eisele M., Mallon T., Schneider A., Linde K., Allwang C., Joos S., Zipfel S., Schulz S., Rost L., Brenk-Franz K., Szecsenyi J., Nikendei C., Härter M., Gallinat J., König H.H., Fierenz A., Vettorazzi E., Zapf A., Lehmann M. & Kohlmann S. (2024) Clinical effectiveness of patient-targeted feedback following depression screening in general practice (GET.FEEDBACK.GP): An investigator-initiated, prospective, multicentre, three-arm, observer-blinded, randomised controlled trial in Germany. *Lancet Psychiatry,* 11(4), 262–273. doi:10.1016/s2215-0366(24)00035-x

48 Lewis G., Hawton K. & Jones P. (1997) Strategies for preventing suicide, *British Journal of Psychiatry.* 171:351–354

49 World Health Organization. Regional Office for the Western Pacific. (2010). Towards evidence-based suicide prevention programmes. WHO Regional Office for the Western Pacific. https://iris.who.int/handle/10665/207049

50 McLennan J. (2015) Persisting without Evidence is a Problem: Suicide Prevention and Other Well-Intentioned Interventions. *Journal of the Canadian Academy of Child and Adolescent Psychiatry,* 24:2, 131–132

Notes

51 National Suicide Prevention Adviser. (2020) Connected and Compassionate: Implementing a national whole of governments approach to suicide prevention (Final Advice). Canberra. https://www.mentalhealthcommission.gov.au/nspo/projects/national-suicide-prevention-adviser-final-advice

52 Institute of Medicine (US) Committee on Pathophysiology and Prevention of Adolescent and Adult Suicide; Goldsmith S.K., Pellmar T.C., Kleinman A.M. & Bunney W.E. (eds). (2002) 8. Programs for suicide prevention. in *Reducing Suicide: A National Imperative*. Washington DC: National Academies Press. https://www.ncbi.nlm.nih.gov/books/NBK220931/; American Public Health Association, *The Role of Public Health in Ensuring Healthy Communities*; Delaware Health and Social Services, *Prevention Definitions and Strategies*

53 WHO. (2018) National suicide prevention strategies: progress, examples and indicators. Geneva: World Health Organization; Licence: CC BY-NC-SA 3.0 IGO

54 Baum F., Townsend B., Fisher M., Browne-Yung K., Freeman T., Ziersch A., Harris P. & Friel S. (2020) Creating Political Will for Action on Health Equity: Practical Lessons for Public Health Policy Actors. *International Journal of Health Policy Management*, 11(7), 947–960; Krakouer M. & Georgatos G. (2020) https://nit.com.au/26-03-2020/1051/the-voice-of-suicide-a-cycle-of-poverty-and-government-inaction; American Public Health Association (2014) *The Role of Public Health in Ensuring Healthy Communities*; Delaware Health and Social Services (2024) *Prevention Definitions and Strategies*. https://dhss.delaware.gov/dhss/dsamh/files/pds.pdf

55 Lewis G., Hawton K. & Jones P. (1997) Strategies for preventing suicide. *British Journal of Psychiatry*. 1997 Oct;171:351-4.

56 Postvention Australia. What is postvention? https://postventionaustralia.org/; together to live. What is postvention? Center for Suicide Prevention. https://www.togethertolive.ca/about/postvention/

57 AIHW Suicide & self-harm monitoring https://www.aihw.gov.au/suicide-self-harm-monitoring/data/technical-notes/methods

58 Raven M., Smith A., & Jureidini J. (2017) Suicide and Self-Harm in Australia: Conceptual Map. (Paper presented at the Royal Australian and New Zealand College of Psychiatrists Congress, Adelaide, South Australia, 30 April – 4 May 2017), http://malesuicidepreventionaustralia.com.au/wp-content/uploads/2017/05/Suicide_and_Self_Harm_in_Australia.pdf

59 Public Health Information Development Unit (PHIDU). Social Health Atlases: Maps. (Adelaide: Torrens University Australia), https://phidu.torrens.edu.au/social-health-atlases/maps

60 Public Health Information Development Unit (PHIDU). Social Health Atlases: Maps. (Adelaide: Torrens University Australia), https://phidu.torrens.edu.au/social-health-atlases/maps

61 Public Health Information Development Unit (PHIDU). Notes on the data: Avoidable mortality by selected cause – 0 to 74 years (Adelaide: Torrens University Australia) https://phidu.torrens.edu.au/notes-on-the-data/health-status-disability-deaths/deaths-0-74-avoidable-suicide

62 AIHW Suicide & self-harm monitoring https://www.aihw.gov.au/suicide-self-harm-monitoring/data/populations-age-groups/suicide-indigenous-australians

63 Saar E. & Burgess T. (2016) Intentional Self-Harm Fatalities in Australia 2001–2013. Data Report DR16 – 16 National Coronial Information System', http://malesuicidepreventionaustralia.com.au/wp-content/uploads/2017/01/NCIS-Report-2016_FINAL.pdf; McPhedran S. & De Leo D. (2013) Miseries suffered, unvoiced, unknown? Communication of suicidal intent by men in "rural" Queensland, Australia. *Suicide and Life-Threatening Behavior*: 5, https://doi.org/10.1111/sltb.12041

64 ABS (2021) Causes of Death. https://www.abs.gov.au/statistics/health/causes-death/causes-death-australia/2021

65 ABS (2022) Causes of Death, Australia.https://www.abs.gov.au/statistics/health/causes-death/causes-death-australia/latest-release

66 ABS (2022) Causes of Death, Australia. https://www.abs.gov.au/statistics/health/causes-death/causes-death-australia/latest-release

67 Knox K. (2014) Approaching Suicide as a Public Health Issue. *Annals of Internal Medicine 161*(2), 151–152. doi:10.7326/M14- 0914

68 Batty G.D., Kivimäki M., Bell S., Gale C.R., Shipley M., Whitley E. & Gunnell D. (2018). Psychosocial characteristics as potential predictors of suicide in adults: An overview of the evidence with new results from prospective cohort studies. *Translational Psychiatry, 8*(1). doi:10.1038/s41398-017-0072-8; Morgan A.J., Roberts R., Mackinnon A.J. & Reifels L. (2022) The effectiveness of an Australian community suicide prevention networks program in preventing suicide: A Controlled Longitudinal Study. BMC Public Health, 22(1). doi:10.1186/s12889-022-14331-1; Niederkrotenthaler T., Gunnell D., Arensman E., Pirkis J., Appleby L., Hawton K., John A., Kapur N., Khan M., O'Connor R.C. & Platt S. (2020) Suicide research, prevention, and COVID-19. *Crisis*, 41(5), 321–330. doi:10.1027/0227-5910/a000

69 Australian Institute of Male Health and Studies. (2017) Clarification of Some Key Terms and Definitions in Suicide Prevention. http://aimhs.com.au/cms/uploads/Guidelines_DefinitionsJan17v3.pdf

70 Nordt C., Warnke I., Seifritz E., & Kawohl W. (2015). Modeling suicide and unemployment: a longitudinal analysis covering 63 countries, 2000–11. *Lancet Psychiatry* 2(3): 239, https://doi.org/10.1016/S2215-0366(14)00118-7; Haw C., Hawton K., Gunnell D. & Platt S. (2015). Economic recession and suicidal behaviour: Possible mechanisms and ameliorating factors. *Int J Soc*

Notes

Psychiatry;61(1):73-81. doi:10.1177/0020764014536545; Reeves A., McKee M., Gunnell D., Chang S.S., Basu S., Barr B., & Stuckler D. (2015). Economic shocks, resilience, and male suicides in the Great Recession: cross-national analysis of 20 EU countries. *Eur J Public Health.* 25(3):404-9. doi:10.1093/eurpub/cku168

71 Jureidini J., & McHenry L. (2020) *The Illusion of Evidence-Based Medicine. Exposing the crisis of credibility in clinical research.* Wakefield Press, Adelaide

72 Hengartner M.P. (2017) Methodological flaws, conflicts of interest, and scientific fallacies: Implications for the evaluation of antidepressants' efficacy and harm. *Frontiers in Psychiatry,* 8. https://doi.org/10.3389/fpsyt.2017.00275

73 Moncrieff J., Cooper R.E., Stockmann T., Amendola S., Hengartner M.P., Horowitz M.A. (2023). The serotonin theory of depression: a systematic umbrella review of the evidence. *Molecular Psychiatry,* 28, 3243–3256 https://doi.org/10.1038/s41380-022-01661-0

74 *The Economist.* (2023) How to stop over-medicalising mental health. https://www.economist.com/leaders/2023/12/07/how-to-stop-over-medicalising-mental-health

75 Welsh H.G., Schwartz L.M. & Woloshin S. (2011) Overdiagnosed: Making People Sick in the Pursuit of Health. Boston: Beacon Press; van Dijk W., Faber M.J., Tanke M.A., Jeurissen P.P. & Westert G.P. (2016) Medicalisation and Overdiagnosis: What Society Does to Medicine. *International Journal of Health Policy and Management.* 1;5(11):619–622. doi:10.15171/ijhpm.2016.121

76 Australian Medical Association (AMA). Mental illness and life insurance: What you need to know – a brief guide, https://ama.com.au/sites/default/files/documents/Mental_illness_and_life_insurance_a_brief_guide_FINAL2.pdf; Zurich Mental Health Frequently Asked Questions – How are mental health conditions diagnosed? https://www.zurich.com.au/content/dam/au-documents/advisers/life-insurance/marketing/mental-health-faq.pdf; headspace (2018). How to get a mental health care plan *https://headspace.org.au/explore-topics/for-young-people/mental-health-care-plan/*

77 Dorter J. (2019) The Impact of Psychosocial Factors on Mental Health and their Implications in Life Insurance; Financial Services Council. https://www.fsc.org.au/news/psychosocial-fsc-kpmg

78 Viola S. & Moncrieff J. (2016) Claims for sickness and disability benefits owing to mental disorders in the UK: Trends from 1995 to 2014. *British Journal of Psychiatry Open,* 2(1), 18–24. doi:10.1192/bjpo.bp.115.002246

79 Mazza D., Brijnath B. & Chakraborty S.P. (2018). Clinical guideline for the diagnosis and management of work-related mental health conditions in general practice. Guideline Development Group Melbourne (Australia): Monash University; 2018. Available: https://www.monash.edu/__data/assets/pdf_file/0004/1696702/

Work-Related-Mental-Health-Clinical-Guideline-for-GPs_Digital_Update-2019.09.10.pdf

80 WorkSafe Victoria Mental Injury Support https://www.worksafe.vic.gov.au/mental-injury-support; RACGP Work related mental health conditions https://www.racgp.org.au/clinical-resources/clinical-guidelines/guidelines-by-topic/endorsed-guidelines/diagnosis-and-management-of-work-related-mental-he; Safe Work Australia & Superfriend (2017/2021) Taking Action: A best practice framework for the management of psychological claims in the Australian workers' compensation sector. https://www.safeworkaustralia.gov.au/doc/taking-action-best-practice-framework-management-psychological-claims-australian-workers-compensation-sector

81 TAL Understanding mental health August 06, 2017. https://www.grouphq.tal.com.au/industry-leadership-and-insights/news-and-articles/2017/09/understanding-mental-health-guide

82 Australian College of Applied Professions. (2021) Nationally Representative Survey Of Australian Workers https://www.acap.edu.au/wp-content/uploads/2021/12/Executive-Summary-ACAP-results-002-1.pdf; Acclaimed Workforce. (2022) Data shows 50% of employees are afraid to reveal their mental health issue at work. https://www.acclaimedworkforce.com.au/employers/data-shows-50-of-employees-are-afraid-to-reveal-their-mental-health-issue-at-work

83 Patty A. (2021) Poor understanding of mental health stifles employment. *Sydney Morning Herald*. https://www.smh.com.au/business/workplace/poor-understanding-of-mental-health-stifles-employment-20210628-p584z3.html

84 ABS. 6362.0 – Employer Training Expenditure and Practices https://www.abs.gov.au/ausstats/abs@.nsf/mf/6362.0; Mental Health First Aid Australia. Over 3 million trained – will you be next? https://www.mhfa.com.au/

85 Workplace Mental Health Institute. (2024) Mental Health First Aid Australia. https://www.wmhi.com.au/mental-health-first-aid/

86 Østerud K.L. (2023) Mental illness stigma and employer evaluation in hiring: Stereotypes, discrimination and the role of experience. Sociology of Health and Illness. 45:90–108. doi:10.1111/1467-9566.13544; Hipes C., Lucas J., Phelan J.C., & White R.C. (2016) The stigma of mental illness in the labor market. *Social Science Research*. 56 (2026) 16–25

87 Dorter J. (2019) The Impact of Psychosocial Factors on Mental Health and Their Implications in Life Insurance; Financial Services Council. https://www.fsc.org.au/news/psychosocial-fsc-kpmg; Sebastião V. & Moncrieff J. (2016) Claims for sickness and disability benefits owing to mental disorders in the UK: trends from 1995 to 2014. *BJPsych Open*, 2, 18–24. doi:10.1192/bjpo.bp.115.002246; Life Insurance Industry, Life Insurance Industry Response To: Productivity Commission's Draft Report on the Social &

Notes

Economic Benefits of Improving Mental Health (23 January 2020), https://www.pc.gov.au/__data/assets/pdf_file/0008/250991/sub821-mental-health.pdf

88 Degerman D. (2023) Mental health: it's not always good to talk. *The Conversation.* https://theconversation.com/mental-health-its-not-always-good-to-talk-197951

89 Staiger T., Maja S., Mueller-Stierlin A.S., Kilian R., Beschoner P., Gündel H., Becker T., Frasch K., Panzirsch M., Schmauß M. & Krumm S. (2020) Masculinity and help-seeking among men with depression: A qualitative study. *Frontiers in Psychiatry, 11.* doi:10.3389/fpsyt.2020.599039

90 McPhedran S. & De Leo D. (2013) Miseries suffered, unvoiced, unknown? Communication of suicidal intent by men in "rural" Queensland, Australia. *Suicide and Life-Threatening Behavior: 5,* https://doi.org/10.1111/sltb.12041; Seidler Z., (2019) We tell men to open up more. But are we ready to listen? *Age,* 18 October https://www.theage.com.au/lifestyle/life-and-relationships/we-tell-men-to-open-up-more-but-are-we-ready-to-listen-20191017-p531mg.html

91 Chandler A., (2021) Masculinities and suicide: unsettling "talk" as a response to suicide in men. *Critical Public Health*: 1–10

92 Chandler A., (2021) Masculinities and suicide: unsettling "talk" as a response to suicide in men. *Critical Public Health*: 1–10

Wakefield Press is an independent publishing and
distribution company based in Adelaide, South Australia.
We love good stories and publish beautiful books.
To see our full range of books, please visit our website at
www.wakefieldpress.com.au
where all titles are available for purchase.
To keep up with our latest releases, news and events,
subscribe to our monthly newsletter.

Find us!

Facebook: www.facebook.com/wakefield.press
Twitter: www.twitter.com/wakefieldpress
Instagram: www.instagram.com/wakefieldpress